ROAR
LIKE A LION
...AGAIN

Restoring Men's Health
After 40...or...

Port R. Martin, EdD

ISBN: 1532710631
ISBN 13: 9781532710636

Dedication

This small volume is dedicated to the memory of Robert Liefmann, MD, whose pioneering work in establishing endocrine nutrition balance for rheumatic diseases successfully treated over 15,000 men and women. Although not recognized appropriately during his lifetime, his body of work was far ahead of his time and has yet to be matched by contemporary researchers. It is hoped that the results of his research and clinical successes will soon be made available to those who suffer from arthritis or desire to achieve a healthful hormonal balance.

Contents

Preface

Acknowledgements

References

Preface

This book is the work of an author who has carefully examined numerous research studies and tested the recommendations to ensure that the facts are straight. The information contained herein is as accurate as he could make it, but it should not be considered comprehensive medical advice. That should only be obtained from a knowledgeable physician who is trained in the areas discussed.

The author intends that the reader will gain some personal insights of value to himself in maintaining a high quality of life into his later years. At a time when modern medicine is making tremendous progress through scientific research to attack many medical conditions that affect those over forty years of age, this book is suggesting that an approach concentrating on returning the body to a chemical state more closely associated with young adults might often be a better and safer approach.

The logic behind this methodology is not exactly new. The Chinese were known as early as 1100 A.D. to provide hormones captured through the urine of young adults and processed for use by the elderly, who were reported to appear younger than their chronological ages. Although the specific nature of these substances (hormones) was not identified until centuries later, the results may be just the same.

Doctors who believe in this logic adhere to the thought that we should, whenever possible, only put into the body that which belongs there naturally. In other words, we should avoid "foreign substances" such as drugs unless they are absolutely necessary. This approach emphasizes a combination of bio-identical hormones and specific nutrients to achieve a chemical balance that gives so many young adults their healthiest years. It may well be that establishing this "younger" body chemistry will provide clues for preventing or treating illnesses currently associated with aging populations.

The author hopes the reader will learn a little more about his body so that he can ask specific questions of his medical advisors and make informed decisions as to treatments that should prove to be the most effective with the least possible side effects.

The information in this book is not designed to serve as a replacement for good diagnostic procedures that should include both appropriate laboratory tests, a physical examination and doctor-patient discussions of symptoms. We expect that treatments for patients should be individually developed to meet unique patient needs and that treatment results should be continuously monitored until optimized.

> Treatments for patients should be individually developed and continuously monitored by trained physicians. One size does not fit all.

And, regardless of the initial results, this approach must follow the patient throughout his life with appropriate adjustments being made as time progresses. Although the techniques discussed may encourage a more youthful appearance and medical profile, aging will continue and body needs will change.

The reader is wished well on this personal voyage with the hope he will find the medical assistance needed to take full advantage of this information.

1

It Happens With Age

It happens every day. We get older. When we are young and waiting for our next birthday, it is an exciting time. However, as the birthdays seem to come closer and closer together, we stop waiting to get older and start remembering when we were young and filled with all the energy and spirit of youth.

This is the time when we start to see some physical changes that may start with a little extra weight around the middle or attached to our backside. We may have some difficulty sleeping all night as trips to the restroom become more and more frequent. We may note some times when we feel unusually warm, hot flushes (flashes) they are called, something we thought only our spouse needed to experience.

Life becomes a bit more challenging as our work responsibilities grow, but we often seem to struggle to maintain the level of intensity that once seemed so natural. We exercise, but the effort to keep our physical appearance looking its best seems to take more and more time…with sometimes less than perfect results.

We have encountered andropause, an experience unknown to us until now and largely not discussed with anyone we know. We may have watched a lady encounter her own surprises as she approached menopause, but that couldn't happen to us, could it? The answer is an emphatic yes! And for the very same reasons, the answer is yes. We are beginning to experience the effects of a change in hormone levels that will affect almost every man who lives to middle age.

This time of change may well occur during the same ages as menopause greets women—between 45 and 55 years of age—but it may affect some individuals earlier or later. We are all unique humans. It is a natural happening that cannot be avoided and is very individual in nature as to the manner it affects each person. One size does not fit all, but there are some common "symptoms" of this condition that we should note.

These symptoms include a loss of strength, decreased energy and increased fatigue, weight gain in the abdominal area, difficulty sleeping through the night, depression, a decreased ability to recover from injuries or exercise, and osteoporosis, a weakening of our bones. There can be a loss of libido and the related erectile dysfunction. The combination of some or all of these symptoms is often reflected in a declining physical appearance and less enjoyment of life in general.

The lion of our youth seems to have disappeared gradually as we have aged. We often prefer sleeping to the roaring of our younger days. No more dancing after scoring a touchdown for us!

Until recently these symptoms were simply ignored by most men and their doctors. It was called "aging," and we all were condemned to do it. Since most of our physicians had no real solution to this naturally occurring process, they could do little but provide help with some of the symptoms, usually in the form of prescription drug products available on the pharmacists' shelves. These products might make the symptoms more tolerable but usually did not address the causes of those symptoms.

We cannot simply stop the aging process at this time although genetic and stem cell research may someday give us all some new approaches. Until that time we must use commonly available means. Most frequently we will be directed to eat nutritious food in modest quantities to control our weights, exercise regularly and then rely on our healthcare providers when illness strikes. This "disease management" system has been in place for many years and is the accepted way to age. But is this the only solution?

There is a new approach to this seemingly inevitable and even threatening aging process. Lost over the years to medical training and research is the value of maintaining proper hormone levels as a hedge against developing the many symptoms that lead us, eventually, to the loss of health and end of our lives. These final steps are often preceded by many years of declining health, a reduced quality of life and severe restrictions on our daily activities.

Currently known as "anti-aging medicine," this new approach has a very solid and simple logic associated with it. Since most of us experienced our healthiest years when we were in our twenties and thirties, this methodology works to re-establish our body chemistries at the levels associated with healthy individuals in that age period. The belief is that proper hormone levels (along with a variety of other chemical properties that should be maintained within established limits) will provide the best opportunities for continuing good health as we enter middle and old ages.

Many of the diseases that are associated with "old age" are closely tied to or associated with a decline in hormone levels. It would seem that restoring these younger and healthy hormone levels might have a positive impact on aging men (and women).

Anti-aging medicine seeks to maintain our health by maintaining our body chemistries—to include hormones—in a healthy range as we grow older.

This is a significantly different approach to health care, one that works to maintain healthy bodies so as to resist the many complications that age can bring. The logic assumes that a healthy body will include a strong immune system which will resist externally and internally encountered threats. It may also prevent some genetic changes, which are brought on by changing chemical conditions, from occurring. Illnesses regularly associated with elderly men and women might well be avoided or at least reduced in effect. The reader (or medical professional) should always be asking the question "Why now?"

"Why didn't this medical challenge occur when I was younger? What was different then that made me so much healthier?"

So why haven't you heard about these solutions before? Bombarded by advertisements for the latest medications, those of us without significant medical educations cannot discern the wheat from the chaff. We are most commonly exposed only to study results that support existing or new products developed by the pharmaceutical industry. Our television sets are filled during the prime viewing hours with solutions for our shortness of breath, weakened bones, overactive bladders and lack of sexual interest or performance. For many of us this is the extent of our medical education and serves to associate specific symptoms with the advertised products' solutions.

But doesn't our family physician have the right information? He or she, too, faces many of the same dilemmas: scattered studies with conflicting results, products promoted by their manufacturers, journals reflecting only those results published by the existing health establishment and an educational process largely dominated by the manufacturers of healthcare products. It is capitalism at its most effective marketing best but not necessarily most helpful form so as to serve our healthcare system.

Limitations may also be placed on physicians by the healthcare organization or insurance systems within which they practice. If they do not have medicines to treat particular symptoms, they must not exist or the symptoms must be tolerated as part of "growing old." Decisions are made as to which drugs or supplements will be available within their organizations, and they often omit significant appropriate hormone products. For those patients without the financial means to go outside their healthcare system, only those limited products are often available.

This book will start with a brief discussion of hormones and their effects on the human body. Then we will venture through a number of topics that should be the concern of every aging man. Many of them will be common to the reader. We hope the insights provided here will encourage all men to look more carefully for help in making the second half of their lives as positive as the first half. Then in the next-to-last chapter we will give you some ideas where to get the physician-guided help you will need to address the issues discussed.

We salute the lion of your youth and hope that the suggestions in this book will bring out his roar once more!

2

Hormones

When complex organisms evolved beyond their single-cell origins, groups of cells became specialized to perform specific functions. This increased complexity required that the cells or groups of cells be able to coordinate their activities to maximize the performance of the new organism. In the human body, two general methods for this communication function dominate: the nervous system and the hormonal system.

To differentiate the two in general terms, the nervous system uses electrical signals to effect signaled needs and the hormonal system uses chemical means. Without either of these systems the human body would have difficulty surviving in a dangerous external environment. Life as we know it would be impossible.

The endocrine system produces hormones which balance the various minerals in our bodies, promote a healthy immune system to fight diseases, encourage and permit adequate sleep, deal with stressful situations, control our internal body temperatures, provide for our sex drive (or libido) and perform hundreds of other functions. Among these many hormones are pregnenolone, estrogens, progesterone, testosterone, dyhydroepiandosterone (DHEA), cortisol, adrenaline, thyroid, human growth hormone and melatonin.

Many of these just mentioned hormones—to include estrogens, testosterone, progesterone and DHEA—are manufactured by the body starting with cholesterol, a substance provided by the liver and through diet. When the body senses that any of these hormones are not being maintained at a healthy level to meet the body's needs, the liver produces more cholesterol so that there is enough to produce the needed hormone or hormones.

This simple act of producing cholesterol as a starting point for the production of one or more of these hormones illustrates a simple diagnostic point. Without testing the patient for all of the possible hormone shortages, it may well be impossible to tell which hormones might need replacement or augmentation. In the manufacturing process, the body can convert the most basic products such as pregnenolone into either progesterone or DHEA. From progesterone, the body may produce testosterone or one of the three human estrogens (estrone, estradiol or estriol). Each individual is different and the impact of our genes is only now beginning to reveal the complexity and differences of each of us.

If the cholesterol cannot be used by the body, it may begin to accumulate in blood vessels, thereby becoming a risk factor for heart-related and other problems. Another way of looking at this issue is to state that cholesterol and proper hormone levels *may* have an inverse relationship. If everything is working properly, as one rises, the other will fall.

> If everything is working properly, cholesterol and hormone levels may be inversely related. If hormone levels are healthy, cholesterol levels will normally be also.

For the purposes of this book we will discuss three types of hormones: natural, synthetic and bio-identical. (These names are not actually entirely correct, but our use of these terms is to distinguish among the three variants.) As one might expect, natural hormones are the ones manufactured by the human body as discussed above.

The term "synthetic hormones" will be used to identify hormones that are manufactured through a pharmaceutical process to closely resemble the natural ones. They differ only slightly and may produce effects within the body that are close, but not necessarily identical, to the natural ones.

Bio-identical hormones are just that, identical at the molecular level in every way to the natural hormones produced by the human body. The hormone receptors in the body will recognize them in the same way as if they were naturally present in the human body. They will usually impact on the cholesterol producing aspect of the liver as if the body was producing them. (These bio-identical hormones may be manufactured from plant or non-human animal materials so they are technically synthetic also.)

There are over 100 hormones produced naturally by a healthy human body. It should also be noted that men and women have exactly the same hormones, but they are in different quantities and may perform similar or different tasks in the two genders. Some of the functions they perform fight stress, maintain the proper level of blood sugar, prevent fatigue and relieve depression. They affect the libido in both sexes and foster proper brain functioning and immune responses.

If bio-identical hormones are available to replace natural hormones which are not at proper levels, one might ask why there is a need for synthetic ones that vary in impact from the natural ones. The answer is quite simple. Naturally occurring substances cannot be patented, and pharmaceutical companies rely on patents to protect their marketing rights after spending hundreds of millions of dollars developing and testing drug products.

Interestingly, several bio-identical and synthetic hormones are produced from the same beginning materials: soy beans and Mexican yams. Those substances are then chemically changed into an intermediate chemical known as *diosgenin*, which can be further converted without great effort into almost any steroid hormone, bio-identical or not (synthetic).

Because of their ability to be patented, synthetic hormones have been the area of concentration for the pharmaceutical firms. Bio-identical products have probably received significantly less emphasis because of the belief that only patented products would prove to be highly profitable. To date this is most likely true.

Although the Chinese were able to utilize products that contained hormones over 1000 years ago, the more modern history of hormones might be traced to the discovery of the testosterone molecule in the early 1930s. Also in the 1930s estrogens and progesterone were identified. In the search for products that could be patented, the pharmaceutical companies moved away from bio-identical products toward those with slightly altered molecular structures.

In 1993 the National Institutes of Health (NIH) began a study of hormone use in women known as the Women's Health Initiative. The study included only synthetic hormones and was stopped abruptly in July 2002 when adverse events were noted within the study. The termination of this study led to the cancellation of a planned parallel study of testosterone replacement in men. Not only have further studies on a large scale not been completed, bio-identical products were not included in the women's study and remain to be studied on a large scale.

In recent years Ms Suzanne Somers has been instrumental in making women conscious of the need to examine their hormone levels and to consider replacement options focused on bio-identical products and nutritional supplements. Unfortunately this same attention has not been focused on men, whose hormone levels also decline with age, causing many of the same symptoms as experienced by women.

3

Physical Appearance

Just as we noted earlier, we get older every day. With that aging our physical appearance slowly changes, and we may lose that physical appearance that we so enjoyed when we were younger. We may think of ourselves as "distinguished" or "showing the signs of becoming an elder," but we are definitely showing the signs of age. Gone are the youthful glow, strong muscles, strong bones and skin elasticity.

Although recent research is showing that telomeres, a short segment of material within cells, may well control the aging of our cells, current technologies have not presented humans with an effective or low cost method of stopping the aging process. This may well change in the future, but for the time we are stuck with our bodies as they grow older. But isn't there some way to help maintain our physical appearance as it was when we were young…or at least younger? The answer may well lie with a balanced approach to maintaining proper hormone levels in our bodies.

Many of us find maintaining a healthy weight is more and more problematic as we get older. Being careful to pay attention to our diets and then eating healthy portions is certainly a start. Combining this with regular exercise is also important. However, as we move into our middle years—45-55 for our purposes—some of these ideas that seemed to work are no longer as effective as they used to be. Many of us see a slow growth of weight around our waistlines, weight that leads us to larger pant sizes and longer belts. Starving ourselves and exercising at excessive levels doesn't seem to show the results we would like.

Here hormones can be the culprit, adding another important factor to weight control. Insulin acts to control blood sugar levels, allowing fat cells to remove excess blood sugar and store it as fat tissue. As we age, both testosterone and progesterone, which help to balance the effects of insulin, decline. This allows insulin to dominate the blood sugar process and create more and more fat. This can ultimately lead to Type II diabetes as well as a figure dominated by excess body fat. For those experiencing this unwanted expansion of waistlines (or fat build-ups in other areas), testing and treatment by a doctor trained in managing hormone levels can be very helpful.

How about wrinkles? Once acquired, they will probably remain unless removed during a cosmetic or surgical procedure. However, maintaining healthy levels of estrogens, testosterone and growth hormone may keep the underlying tissues healthy and strong. These hormones boost the manufacture of collagen and elastin as well as hydration of the skin. Loss of elastin allows the gradual stretching of the skin into those wrinkles that mark us as old. Therefore, these hormones may help skin age more slowly.

We also may be able to control or even restore hair on our heads by using appropriate hormones. This should be done carefully, however, to ensure that secondary effects in other parts of our bodies with negative impacts do not occur. To some degree, hair color may be maintained or improved by ensuring that ACTH (adrenocorticotrope hormone) levels are appropriate.

Are the arm muscles looking a little limp? How about the backs of your arms? Sometimes even exercise, weight lifting as an example, can't maintain the type of fitness that we like to see. In men this is often an indicator that testosterone and/or DHEA levels are low. Human growth hormone may also be a factor, but testosterone is needed by all of us to maintain strong, healthy muscle tissue. As with all hormone-related conditions, however, one should not jump to an immediate conclusion that low testosterone is the cause. Proper testing and interpretation of the results by a trained physician is the key to getting things headed in the right direction.

> Testing hormone levels and interpretation of the results by a trained physician is the place to start when looking to improve muscle tone and strength.

And speaking of muscles, the heart is no exception. There are more testosterone receptor sites on the heart than on any other organ. A weak heart can lead to difficulty doing most tasks; even walking can become a problem. Strengthening the heart can help improve exercise performance, and that can lead to a healthier overall appearance. (There is also some evidence that supplemental testosterone may help patients recover from congestive heart failure.)

On a more general level, we appear healthier and energetic if we feel well. Establishing a healthy style of living to include proper hormone levels, nutrition appropriate to our needs and exercise to keep all body parts functioning regularly can work together to keep our bodies feeling well. We will reflect that health in our appearance.

4

Strength

Men usually have about 50 percent more muscle mass than women. This is associated with an increase in strength as well. As young adults, men demonstrate and maintain this added strength naturally as testosterone routinely contributes to the regular maintenance of muscle tissue. As they age, however, men see their testosterone levels slowly fall at an average rate of 1 to 2 percent per year, starting in their early thirties.

We are all probably familiar with athletes who "lose a step or two" as they get older. We consider this a natural happening even though a few lucky ones seem to be "ageless" and participate at a high level far longer than their contemporaries. Although all men can expect their testosterone levels and related muscular performance to fall, it is not on a schedule that treats everyone equally. If any man lives long enough, he will eventually see declining performance from a muscular standpoint.

For those who are not professional athletes but to whom exercise is a regular habit, they will see a gradual decline in performance within their chosen exercise routine. Longer exercise periods and more effort will not correct the problem as the body is no longer able to create and maintain muscle tissue to the same level as that of a healthy 25-year-old. What is the aging, health-focused man to do?

The answer is not as simple as it might seem since hormones do not act in a vacuum. They routinely interact with other hormones and are affected by the overall needs of the human body. Should one hormone be at an inappropriate level, the body will act to correct the problem and that may affect another function or associated hormone level(s).

As an example, we should examine the possible impact of declining testosterone on the prostate. Why? It is simply because a very large number of men, perhaps as high as 85%, will die with prostate cancer. Although it may not spread beyond the prostate nor be the cause of death, it will be present.

Here is how this may well happen. As we age, many hormone levels will decline as determined by genetic and environmental causes. Among those that commonly decline (just as testosterone does) is progesterone. Yes, progesterone. Although it is often associated with women, both genders have the same hormones although they are at different levels and may have different functions.

Progesterone in men acts to help balance the impact of insulin. As men age and progesterone levels fall, men often begin to gain weight around the midsection. This added weight—mostly fat tissue—demonstrates that insulin is not properly balanced by adequate progesterone levels. Insulin acts to maintain proper blood sugar levels and stores the excess sugar as fat. When insulin begins to dominate the process because of low progesterone, fat levels rise.

Fat cells, through a process known as aromatization, can convert testosterone to estradiol, one of the two strongest estrogens. Estradiol has been linked to at least six cancers in women, including in the tissue that has the same fetal origins as the male prostate. Although this link has not been conclusively proven, it has a very logical basis.

As fat around the middle begins to grow, this process can convert more and more testosterone to estradiol, increasing the risk of prostate cancer while denying men's bodies further of the testosterone needed for healthy muscle and bone tissues. If nothing is done to counteract this process, strength will continue to decline and reduced activity levels will result. This further aggravates the situation.

As you can see from this example, restoring and balancing men's hormones to optimal levels requires attention to all hormones, not just testosterone. If restoring an adequate testosterone level is not enough to address this condition, how should it be approached? The answer lies in a comprehensive view that includes guidance by a trained medical professional assisted by laboratory testing, physical examination and patient interviewing. Testing can verify specific hormone levels, but only the patient can accurately relate the symptoms that he is experiencing. Also, only a doctor trained to interpret the results in the context of the patient's symptoms and physical examination can accurately recommend a treatment regimen. Together these aspects provide the first part of the answer.

Once a treatment plan is established, it must be monitored to ensure that it is working properly. Each person is an individual, and his body will respond in a unique manner. Adjustments to hormones and other supplements provided should be anticipated until the best possible results are established. This approach also may determine that some other cause must be treated.

For all too long, a gradual loss of strength has been a commonly accepted companion of aging. Although it may seem natural to those who have not received treatment, men are no longer required to lose their ability to enjoy activities that require muscular activity simply because they are elderly. The lion can, indeed, roar again!

But it may not take a wheel chair existence or tottering walk to indicate a need for improving muscular strength. The condition known familiarly as incontinence (or urinary incontinence) may well be a strong indication that muscle strength is waning. Addressed by a number of drug products, the inability of men to refrain from frequent trips to the restroom, often continuing all night long, can be frustrating and fatiguing.

The solution may be as simple as raising testosterone levels to a proper level and then exercising the muscles that control urination. Known as the Kegel maneuver, these exercises simply target the weakened muscles by starting and then stopping urination. In a week or so in combination with an adequate testosterone level, these simple exercises can eliminate the need to urinate constantly. Want to enjoy a few beers at the football game without multiple trips to the men's room? Give this simple solution a try. All you need is a doctor's prescription for a proper dose of testosterone and some exercise time, which can be captured almost anywhere.

Establishing a proper level of testosterone and the related strengthening of muscles may well extend your time in the stands and away from the restroom lines.

Are you concerned with wrinkles and that exterior evidence of aging? Maintaining proper muscle strength can keep the muscle layer just below the skin strong and tight...just as it was when you were young. This is a preventative action and probably will not remove wrinkles once they have formed. That will require the assistance of your doctor, a variety of products applied internally or externally to the skin or your favorite plastic surgeon.

Wherever muscles are involved, proper hormone levels are needed to maintain or improve strength. What about one of the strongest and most important muscles in the body—the heart? Here too, proper hormone levels can keep or improve cardiac function. Although the evidence is not available through large-scale clinical trials, some small studies show that testosterone supplementation for those recovering from congestive heart failure may benefit patients.

Weight lifters and professional athletes for many generations have taken doses of testosterone or testosterone-like substances way above those needed for normal strength and good overall health. This abuse has given a bad reputation for those of us with normal hormonal needs. Don't let abuse discourage proper use. Ensure that you establish a proper physiologic dose with your doctor, and the resulting improvements may be noted throughout your body.

Once optimum levels have been obtained, however, monitoring should continue. There is evidence to demonstrate that over time reduced supplementation may be appropriate or changes in other hormone levels will require modified doses. This is a lifetime task, not a one-time fix.

5

Energy

Fatigue is a common complaint of those whose hormones are not in a properly balanced state. It might be only one hormone or it could be a combination of hormones that is causing the problem as the different hormones often act in concert with each other.

Low thyroid hormone should be considered by physicians when the fatigue is primarily present when you first wake up. Being active can make this condition less obvious, and this form of fatigue will often disappear after arising and becoming active.

Another possible cause of fatigue is low blood sugar, a condition that may occur when insulin is not properly balanced with progesterone. This type of fatigue will most often occur in the afternoon. This may also become a problem when driving a car for a significant period of time.

Personal Story...

The author has always had problems with fatigue when driving a car for any length of time. His remedy of choice was Coca Cola®, to be consumed mostly on the first day of long trips and in significant quantities. With his balanced hormones, probably progesterone and testosterone being the primary ones, driving without fatigue is a pleasure. The soft drink complete with caffeine can stay in the refrigerator at home along with the extra calories.

Depression may also be linked to fatigue and a progesterone shortfall. By adding progesterone, the insulin level can be stabilized, and the brain will be getting sufficient sugar to remain alert.

In men low testosterone can be a cause of fatigue, especially during periods of intense physical activity but also during a routine workday. This type of fatigue will be present all through the day and will bring on a desire to rest or resist activity of any sort. Low DHEA may cause the same symptoms. With this type of fatigue, growing inactivity will lead to a further loss of muscle strength and a general decline in ability to use the muscles affected.

An inadequate level of human growth hormone (HGH) can also leave one feeling fatigued. This may be a mild condition during the day but become more evident late in the day. This hormone is important for tissue growth and repair so it may be very important to those who exercise to any extreme. HGH is sometimes used as an anti-aging treatment but can only legally be prescribed for a proven adult HGH deficiency syndrome. However, since the body is no longer growing as during youthful years, there must be some concern expressed for potential side effects that excess HGH might encourage. Careful monitoring by a physician should be exercised.

Inadequate levels of thyroid, progesterone, DHEA, cortisol, HGH and testosterone can all cause feelings of fatigue. One should always use testing to establish the cause and then prescribe appropriate bio-identical hormone products.

A potassium shortage may occur if the body does not have a sufficient quantity of human growth hormone. Since potassium is critical to the proper functioning of cells, proper levels of HGH might need to be restored by treatment to resolve this issue.

As with many physical problems, proper nutrition can be a factor in fatigue or lack of energy. For instance, eating foods with a high sugar content can provide a burst of energy when first eaten, but there is usually a rapid decline in energy level shortly after the boost. This occurs because insulin may address the rise in sugar or sweet-tasting by responding in too large a degree. The "sugar high" is well known and may encourage over eating when blood sugar levels fall below adequate levels. "Diet drinks" are often treated by the body the same as those containing sugar, thereby leading some to the same high-sugar-low-sugar roller coaster effect.

Among supplements, vitamin B_{12} can help to provide energy while assisting in the development of red blood cells. These cells are critical in carrying sufficient quantities of oxygen throughout the body, thereby assisting in the processing of glucose for fuel. Magnesium and iron are also helpful in ensuring that the body has sufficient energy. However, iron in excess can negatively affect men's health so monitoring by a physician is a must.

One additional supplement may be critical in keeping energy levels high: Coenzyme Q10 (CoQ10). For those who are taking statin drugs to lower cholesterol, this supplement is absolutely necessary as these drugs are known to remove available CoQ10 from the body. CoQ10 helps to ensure strong blood flow through the heart and to maintain healthy muscles. CoQ10 can be depleted by many other prescription drugs as well so this should be monitored for all patients.

There are many other nutritional elements that can play a role in maintaining adequate energy. If a deficiency may be at least partially to blame for low energy, consultation with a healthcare professional skilled in nutrition is a must. Even better is to find one who also understands the need to optimize hormones at the same time.

> The guidance of a trained nutritional expert who understands the similar importance of balancing hormones can be invaluable.

Stress can call upon the body to have extra energy available to deal with a crisis. To assist this effort, the adrenal glands release stored reserves of cortisol, a hormone which then guides the release of sugar so that the brain and important muscles have the extra energy they need. This hormone is critical for addressing stress, and its absence will lead to increasing levels of fatigue.

The importance of cortisol should be noted here. Recurring periods of stress or even single catastrophic events can cause adrenal fatigue. This may be one of the results that is reflected in Post Traumatic Stress Disorder (PTSD), most commonly associated with military troops who experience stressful situations in combat. However, this is even more common in daily life when chaotic situations repeat themselves and challenging situations occur. A prolonged period of stress may lead to a decreased ability of the adrenal glands to secrete adequate levels of cortisol. This then becomes a major cause of fatigue.

There is one last factor that must be evaluated: sleep. If the body does not get adequate levels of sleep, the lack of rest will be demonstrated by a feeling of fatigue during the day. Melatonin levels that are sufficient will allow the body to lose less energy during the night by reducing cortisol levels that are effective during the day but not needed at night. Melatonin also can help in the release of HGH so that the body can store more energy for the following day and the production of thyroid hormone (T_3) so that waking up refreshed is common.

6

Osteoporosis

As we age, we become less able to maintain healthy bones naturally. Although women may appear to be more vulnerable to the progressive disease of osteoporosis, men may also encounter this condition. In the case of men, they may be older than women when they first encounter this weakening of the skeletal system because of the heavier nature of men's bones in early adulthood. As many as 25% of men over the age of 60 will encounter a fracture brought on by osteoporosis as compared to 50% of all women. Although this is, perhaps, less threatening to men, it is still serious for those 25% who suffer broken bones.

Before we look at the impact of osteoporosis, we should examine how the human body can naturally maintain healthy bones as it does during most of our early adult years. Two types of cells are associated with the natural renewal of our bone structure: osteoclasts and osteoblasts.

Osteoclasts have two primary functions in this process. First they remove old bone tissue that no longer is in optimum condition. The old bone tissue is not simply discarded but the minerals, particularly calcium, are then made available for use elsewhere in the body. After they remove the old and often brittle bone, the osteoclasts leave behind a lattice framework to help support the replacement bone tissue.

The next step in this process has the osteoblasts attaching the new bone to this lattice framework, somewhat as plaster is applied to a wire screen to achieve maximum strength. If the osteoblasts were to apply the new tissue without this lattice work, the new bone would not be of optimum strength.

As many of us age, the osteoclasts continue working but at a pace that the osteoblasts cannot match. This creates an imbalance in the bone renewal process, meaning that more old bone is being removed than can be replaced by the new bone.

Bones encountering this condition become less strong or more "porous" from the vacant areas thus created. As the bones are weakened, they become more likely to fracture from a variety of causes. Even minor stresses such as walking or bumping into an object may cause bones with osteoporosis to break.

The exact cause of this imbalance between osteoclasts and osteoblasts has not been clearly defined, but it is apparently associated with reduced levels of key hormones in both men and women as we age. Because of this in the past, osteoporosis was a reason for women to begin taking supplemental estrogen. However, in 1999 the FDA eliminated this reason for prescribing estrogen purely on the basis of a diagnosis of osteoporosis.

So, how does one know that osteoporosis is present? There is a process using DEXA (dual-energy X-ray absorptionometry) scans to note the difference between the existing bone density being measured and that of a 24-year-old individual. In addition there are several other methods, including a special type of CT scan and ultrasound. A condition known as osteopenia precedes osteoporosis and is an indication that the process of bone weakening is underway.

Once a diagnosis of osteoporosis has been established, action by the patient is required to reestablish proper bone health. For many years supplemental estrogen and increased calcium intake were prescribed for women. More recently a class of drugs known as bisphosphonates has been prescribed with some possible serious consequences.

These drugs—under a number of names such as Fosamax®, Boniva®, Actonel® and Reclast®—work to stop the osteoclasts from removing old bone tissue but also from establishing the lattice required by the osteoblasts to complete their part of the bone renewal process. These drugs also have a long half-life, meaning that they remain in the body for many years after they are no longer used by a patient and continue to work as designed.

The use of these drugs may present a partial indication of bone formation when treatment first begins. This might be explained by simply noting that the osteoclasts are no longer removing the old bone and some osteoblast deposits of new bone material continue. However, the new bone does not have the strength that once marked healthy, young bones since the osteoclast-provided lattice is not present. The end result is bones that may look slightly more dense to a

DEXA scan but which are notably less strong because of the lack of the structurally supportive lattice work.

A second potentially negative impact may result from the lack of routine bone maintenance that once kept our bones healthy. We humans are constantly stressing our bones when we jar them, bear weight on them or bump into objects. These "minor" bone injuries in the healthy adult are then repaired by the available osteoclasts and osteoblasts working normally. Without the work of the osteoclasts, these small bone injuries or minor fractures may remain improperly healed. These minute fractures then provide stress areas in the vicinity of those places where they may build up slowly and reinforce each other. The result can be what appears to be spontaneous fracture with no identifiable cause other than a minor trip or bump.

Should a fracture occur from the presence of osteoporosis or some other cause, the fractured area will have difficulty healing properly without significant surgical interventions when significant amounts of the bisphosphonate drugs mentioned earlier are still present. Even if some healing occurs, the resulting new bone tissue may not be nearly as strong as a normal healing process would dictate.

So what should the patient with osteoporosis or osteopenia identified actually do? No action is a poor solution as the loss of bone density can be expected to continue at a rate dictated by individual physical characteristics. Are the bisphosphonates the only available solution? If so, every patient should be prepared for a variety of potential side effects, many similar to those already associated with osteoporosis and the loss of bone density with an associated structural strength reduction.

Luckily there is a growing body of evidence that indicates that the normal process by which humans maintain strong bones can be restored by simply achieving a proper balance of steroid hormones as would be found in healthy young adults. For many years women were treated with estrogens, but, as noted earlier in this chapter, the FDA has been presented with evidence that this is not necessarily an effective treatment. Ensuring proper nutrition and participating in weight-bearing exercise have also been routinely prescribed.

It would appear that progesterone (not progestins) might be the answer. Dr. John R. Lee, a Northern California family physician, noted significant bone density gains in his female patients who were using bio-identical progesterone. Although his research did not prove the value of progesterone to the extent of a significantly larger scientific study, the trend he saw was, and remains, well-worth considering when a treatment plan is designed for a patient.

In addition, the hormones testosterone and DHEA (dyhydroepiandrosterone) are known to assist men in developing new bone. Both of these hormones are known to decline steadily in men as they age, leading to the conclusion that supplementary amounts of these two hormones might well assist in addressing the needs of a male patient diagnosed with osteopenia or osteoporosis.

Since hormones are known to interact with each other and have both complementary and opposing interactions, the argument can be advanced that treatments should include both an analysis of the patients overall hormone levels and appropriate treatment to bring them to a balance for a healthy individual, who is then less likely to have bone-related issues. This further argues for standards to be established that are closer to those of young adults than those currently associated with age-related peers. If bone density is compared to that of a 24-year-old, then hormone levels should be as well.

In addition certain supplements may be helpful in building new bone. These should, in a similar manner, be prescribed as needed following an analysis of the patient's identified needs following appropriate tests. Simply taking multiple vitamins and other supplements without a sound basis is not likely to achieve maximum results.

In any case, if the osteoclasts and osteoblasts are not doing their jobs in replacing old bone with the new, other actions will likely not have much effect. As discussed earlier, bisphosphonates stop the osteoclasts from removing the old bone tissue and preparing the areas for osteoblasts to deposit the new bone materials. Adding more calcium in whatever form to a patient's treatment regime may benefit other body functions, but it will not result in new or stronger bones. The entire process must work in concert to achieve the desired results.

Once the bone renewal process has been reestablished, such aspects as proper diet, exercise, and supplementary vitamins and minerals may enhance new bone development. In addition to calcium and vitamin D, both well-known to be needed for proper bone health, strontium, vitamin K2, copper, zinc, magnesium, selenium and several other nutrients may be helpful. Consultation with a knowledgeable physician should guide a patient's choices. The author believes that only those supplements that establish a natural environment for good bone health should be chosen. More is not always better, and large doses of calcium have proven to be harmful in some studies.

Once the natural bone renewal process has been reestablished and the appropriate vitamins and minerals are available to support the reconstruction effort, weight-bearing exercise may assist in building strong bones with a healthful density. The human body is amazingly adaptable and will strengthen those areas where stresses are noted. Exercises that strengthen muscles will also demand that the supporting bone structures be strong.

Healthy bone renewal must involve the teamwork of osteoclasts and osteoblasts to be effective.

Once the renewal process is established, some vitamins, minerals and exercise may be important.

Bisphosphenates should be used with caution and full knowledge of the possible side effects.

7

Depression

As men encounter andropause, it is not unusual for them to develop symptoms of depression at that time. The loss of energy discussed in Chapter 5 is quite possibly related to the same cause. In many men these symptoms are the result of a low testosterone level, and a return to normal levels of that hormone alone may restore overall physical strength and an improved outlook on life. Fatigue can be a cause of depression, and depression can be a cause of fatigue. A loss of libido at the same time depression is encountered is another indication that a low testosterone level is the primary cause.

Some other symptoms of depression can be a lack of interest in activities previously enjoyed, a lack of self-confidence, a lack of motivation or ambition to do things or even a lack of enjoyment of life itself.

When investigating solutions for this, several aspects should be kept in mind. First, normal levels of testosterone may not be the best levels for all men. In other words we are all individuals, and our bodies function best with hormone levels that are somewhat unique to ourselves. A testosterone level that is adequate for one individual may well be too low or too high for another. Doctors treating a patient must blend laboratory normal values with the reports by the patient as to results.

Second, it is important to realize that a single hormone may not be the cause—or at least sole cause—of a specific condition. As noted earlier, our bodies contain over one hundred types of hormones, and their levels and actions interact with each other. Achieving the proper level of one hormone may drive one or more others from an optimum point. This may challenge both the doctor and the patient in trying to achieve the most helpful balance of all hormones.

The hormone progesterone also may well have a positive impact on men suffering from depression. It is a natural antidepressant and may reach lower than optimum levels at the same time that the effects of low testosterone are first noted by a patient. The human body can also internally make testosterone from progesterone; therefore, an external source of progesterone may raise testosterone levels almost simultaneously.

As men and women age, progesterone levels steadily decline until they become significantly low at about the time men can expect to encounter andropause. Although this age may fall most commonly in the 45 to 55 age bracket, individuals may encounter this issue either before or after this point.

By the time most men are 50 to 60 years of age, their bodies will usually have significantly low progesterone. When this occurs, insulin may begin to dominate a careful balance with progesterone that is needed to maintain proper blood sugar levels. Men will have a tendency to gain weight in fat in the middle of their bodies. This abdominal fat has a number of negative impacts to include accelerating the decline in testosterone levels.

Fat cells have the ability to convert testosterone to estradiol through an enzyme known as aromatase. At the very time when men are noting the symptoms of reduced testosterone, their bodies are likely to be reducing the available testosterone and increasing the levels of estradiol, a process that may well increase the possibility of developing prostate cancer. This is discussed further in Chapter 10 as type II diabetes is also associated with this fat gain with age.

Another hormone that can assist in preventing depression is thyroid. This type of deficiency may show itself when a man finds himself depressed upon waking in the morning. This particular form of depression can be treated rather quickly by establishing a proper level of thyroid hormone. Low levels of DHEA are also associated with depression, and depression may lessen or disappear as DHEA levels rise.

As one can see from this chapter, achieving a proper hormonal balance can have a life-changing impact to include the improvement of physical and mental health. Testosterone, thyroid, DHEA and progesterone levels should be tested to begin treatment for depressive feelings, especially with those suspected to be related to aging. Then, once treatment has begun, levels must be monitored to ensure that a proper balance of those hormones is maintained and that the levels of other hormones are not impacted negatively.

8

Heart Disease

When the 20th century began, coronary artery disease was rare. As life expectancies have risen, heart disease has become the leading cause of death in the United States. Although heart disease can occur at any age, it becomes a dominant cause of death as age progresses. Interestingly, as we age our hormone levels tend to decrease. Could there be a connection?

Hormones play an important part in maintaining a healthy blood supply to many key organs, and, as this crucial source of nutrients and oxygen becomes restricted, we can expect negative impacts. Many studies have shown that maintaining a healthy balance of hormones can do much to reduce the risk factors associated with heart disease.

Even if you are an outwardly healthy individual who has carefully maintained an appropriate weight while exercising regularly, the slow loss of physical capabilities can be a sign that your cardiovascular system is showing an inability to maintain the needed blood supply to muscles and other organs. If you are tired after climbing a set of stairs, your heart may be "feeling its age." Do regular morning walks seem more fatiguing than they once were? These signs of decreased physical performance could well indicate that your heart is beginning to feel the effects of reduced hormone levels.

Your heart is a large muscle that works 24 hours every day to supply your body with blood where needed. Since testosterone is a key element involved in building and maintaining muscle strength as we discussed in Chapter 4, you would be correct in assuming it is important to heart health. In fact the heart has more receptor sites for testosterone than any other organ. Many studies have shown that low testosterone levels are associated with an increased risk for heart disease.

This type of information may seem to argue for testosterone supplementation when heart disease risks begin to increase, however, the challenge is much more complicated. There are a number of other hormones and issues that can make an easy solution elusive.

Let's start the discussion with cholesterol, a substance that has been linked to heart health by a number of studies. Cholesterol levels tend to rise with age, a possible strong connection to the parallel decline in hormone levels. In fact, cholesterol is the basic substance from which the steroid hormones are made by the body. In the proper forms and amounts it is critical to life. Although we may alter slightly the amount of cholesterol in our bodies, most of it is made internally, some of which may be in response to a need for hormones requiring it as an initial building block.

Rather than treat cholesterol that is not at an appropriate level with drugs that may have significant side effects, it may prove beneficial to provide supplemental hormone(s) so that the body will stop producing the excess cholesterol. Once the proper hormone levels are achieved, the body will, on its own, lower the available cholesterol levels.

High cholesterol levels may be an indication that the body is attempting to manufacture certain hormones.

Personal Story...

The author first was tested for hormone levels in April 2009. When he began treatment in May 2009, his total cholesterol was 232. Testing in August 2009 indicated a reduced level of 165, close to that maintained during his younger years. The only medications received were bio-identical hormone supplements; no cholesterol lowering drugs were used.

If high blood pressure is diagnosed, this may indicate a "plumbing problem," blood vessels that are restricted in some way forcing the heart to increase pressure so as to maintain proper blood flow. Rather than taking drugs to thin the blood or relax the blood vessels, the patient might address this issue by working to create blood vessels that are more open and flexible. Thyroid hormone may assist in achieving this end by making arterial walls more flexible. DHEA can also assist by dilating blood vessels. By driving hormone levels to healthy levels, cholesterol that might be the cause of blockages can be reduced; this may well allow a freer flow of blood with the associated lower blood pressure.

Although it is less common than high blood pressure, low blood pressure could be the result of lower than healthy levels of aldosterone, vasopressin or cortisol. Symptoms of this problem may result in dizziness when standing from a seated or bent-over position or in possessing little resistance to stress. Increasing one or more of these three hormones as indicated by low test levels may well resolve the problem.

Low levels of human growth hormone (HGH) are associated with an increased risk of heart disease and possible death. Since HGH is utilized by adults to maintain or increase muscle mass, it seems logical that it may be related to the maintenance of a strong and healthy heart muscle. Treatment of those who experience low HGH levels with supplementary amounts has shown improvement in heart muscle mass. This, in turn, has led to improved blood flow and the associated gains in patient health.

In addition to those hormones already mentioned in this chapter, an abnormal level of insulin is sometimes associated with cardiovascular problems.

The key aspect of this chapter is to note the important roles that our hormones play in maintaining a healthy cardiovascular system. It is not enough to simply lower cholesterol with a drug or to make dietary changes, but rather the affected individuals must press to discover the cause of the high cholesterol. If it is simply an age-related decline in hormones which is causing levels to rise, perhaps the addition of supplementary hormones will have a very beneficial impact on heart health.

It is important to note that any of the ideas noted in this chapter should be verified by appropriate tests and consultation with a trained physician, one who knows the impact of hormones on heart health and their interactions with each other.

In some cases establishing proper hormone levels may lead to improved cardiovascular health.

9

Libido

One study has shown that 70% of women lose interest in sex and over 50% of men encounter the same lack of interest. This can certainly cause difficulties in any relationship where sexual interest is non-existent with one of the couple. But doesn't Viagra® resolve this problem? The answer is that although the drug (along with several others) is widely touted as a cure for sexual problems, it only addresses the physical aspects of the act, not the mental aspect of interest.

Since this loss of interest seems to occur with advancing age, might there be a connection to decreasing levels of hormones? Most certainly so! And, in this case, the most common hormone involved is the same for both men and women: testosterone. Often thought to be a hormone associated with men, it also has the job of creating sexual interest in women. The aspect of interest is paired with physical arousal so the Viagra®-like drugs can assist in avoiding impotence but may not address interest to any degree.

Yet there may be more to this sexual "equation" than just increasing testosterone. DHEA may be a factor in helping men deal with erectile dysfunction. Even estrogen has been shown to increase desire in animal tests; this may be problematic for some men because of negative side effects relating to the prostate.

Cortisol and human growth hormone (HGH) may also be players here as they can enhance the quality of physical activity.

Although this seems like a simple issue to address at first, one can see that there are, again, a number of hormones involved in sexual activities. First there must be some interest to get things started and then the body must respond to the stimulation that follows.

It is important to note here that both partners should be treated as necessary. Any relationship can be threatened when the interest is not balanced properly. And, as with all hormone treatments, they should be individualized to meet the specific needs of the patient. Simply jumping to a testosterone solution may cause problems that are unrelated to the sexual ones being treated. Also, doses should be in the physiologic range, meaning at levels naturally occurring in the human body. In this case, men will probably require much larger doses than women.

Although testosterone may well be a primary cause of libido loss, other inappropriate hormone levels may be implicated.

10

Diabetes

There are two types of diabetes; both involve the interactions of insulin with the body. The first type, known as Type I, occurs when the pancreas is not capable of producing an adequate amount of insulin. In many cases the pancreas loses the ability to make any insulin at all. This type of diabetes is often common in children and is sometimes known as juvenile diabetes. Those who must deal with this form of diabetes must monitor their blood sugar level constantly and use supplementary insulin to supply that which the body no longer can. At present there are no alternative treatments for this form.

The second form of diabetes, known as Type II, occurs when the body becomes less sensitive to insulin, often leading to excess insulin being secreted by the pancreas to try to overcome the insulin resistance. Blood sugar levels, as with Type I diabetes, must often be monitored manually as the body is not able to use the available insulin properly. In most cases, however, the insulin does continue to work with fat cells, storing increasing amounts of blood sugar in that form. This leads to a growing obesity, which then further complicates the situation.

This form of diabetes often can be addressed by reducing the amount of body fat through exercise and diet, but patients encountering this challenge often find the remedy is not easily achieved. When we are young and have an optimum balance of our natural hormones, we may be able to adjust our weight very effectively by being careful about what we eat, how much we eat, and including adequate exercise in our schedules. However, with age and decreasing hormone levels, the easy solutions of our youth may require assistance.

There are a number of possible hormones that may need adjustment to establish a weight-losing environment. Deficiencies in testosterone and progesterone are possible keys, but cortisol, DHEA, human growth hormone, aldosterone and thyroid levels may also be low. Estradiol, insulin and cortisol may all be high. The correct place to start is to measure these key hormones to have an accurate starting point for adjusting levels to optimums. A physician trained to work with hormones can match the hormone levels with the symptoms reported by the patient.

Testosterone may be in short supply because the fat gained may be converting it to estradiol through a process known as aromatization. This increasing estradiol is believed by some to be the ultimate cause of prostate cancer as that hormone is known to cause cancer in women in the tissues with the same fetal origins as the male prostate. Although testosterone is believed by some to be the cause of prostate cancer, it is quite possibly the conversion of existing testosterone to estradiol that is problematic.

Both testosterone and progesterone may be useful in treating type II diabetes...as determined by testing and examination of other factors.

If testosterone is going to be part of the treatment process, then it might be wise to start by balancing other hormones and beginning the weight loss effort first. In many cases, this might argue for a beginning with progesterone (or other diagnosed shortfalls) and adjusting diet and exercise. Once a proper hormonal balance is established and weight loss has started, testosterone could be added to assist in building muscle as supported by exercise. Progesterone appears to help balance insulin levels and may reduce excess insulin.

Dr. Edward Lichten has reported that low testosterone is associated with most diabetic men. Treatment with testosterone may well reduce cell resistance to insulin, meaning that cells more readily admit glucose. This is exactly what treatment should do in reversing the body's resistance to insulin, a condition leading to an increase in fat. (As discussed earlier, this, in turn, reduces testosterone.) The supplementary testosterone helps reverse the spiral toward increased obesity and insulin resistance.

With life expectancies slowly but steadily increasing, we can expect to see more and more aging men reaching a point where hormone deficiencies are noted. The first step is probably to watch for the telltale growth of body fat around the waist. This sets in play the problems noted earlier in this chapter. A proper treatment regimen would include the monitoring of hormone levels starting at an early age, perhaps 40-45 for most men, so as to avoid the beginning fat gain. Early treatment could readily slow this growing national problem.

11

Bladder and Prostate

These are two organs than most aging men will need to keep under surveillance for unacceptable behavior. For young men these are not a problem, and they pay little attention to them. It is important to note that their testosterone and other hormone levels may be quite high, as high as they may be for most of the rest of their lives. This leads one to believe, as problems start to mount in the aging male, that perhaps declining hormone levels may be the source of some of the challenges presented.

Starting with the bladder, as age increases men may find that they spend significant amounts of time looking for the nearest bathroom. A casual lunch with friends that includes a beer or two also includes three or four trips to the men's room. Delaying these trips to test the local facilities is not an option. Likewise, nary a night passes without numerous trips to relieve oneself. Wouldn't it be nice if one could have a complete night's sleep without these routine trips to the bathroom.

In fact, many men may reduce or eliminate extra trips to empty their bladders simply by increasing the strength of the muscle that once could handle the building pressure with ease. But before the muscle can be strengthened, it will usually need some testosterone to support this added strength. Given in a physiologic dose, testosterone can give the aging male just the boost needed to build strength in this crucial and somewhat embarrassing area.

In combination with supplemental testosterone a simple exercise, known as the Kegel maneuver, will finish the job. This exercise involves beginning urination and then physically stopping the flow, then repeating the exercise multiple times. After 7-10 days of combining testosterone supplementation and this exercise routine, most men can regain control of their bladders without other drugs. This may well require the continuation of testosterone treatment to maintain overall body levels at an appropriate level as a one-time treatment is unlikely to help the older male achieve more than an initial success. In other words, this particular problem is an indication that there is a larger problem which should be treated.

There is one more note of importance relating to bladder health. Low levels of vitamin D are associated with an increased risk of bladder cancer. This vitamin, often associated with achieving appropriate levels of sun exposure, is apparently no longer being made in adequate amounts by many humans. Dark skin is also known to further decrease the body's ability to produce adequate levels of vitamin D. As discussed later in Chapter 13, this particular supplement may be a must for this and many other reasons. As included in multi-vitamin tablets, the dosage is probably too low to provide much value, particularly in combination with the lowered testosterone of the aging male.

Not far geographically from the bladder, the prostate performs its functions. There is a tendency for the prostate to gradually increase in size with age. This seems to parallel the decrease of testosterone in men that is a natural part of the aging process. What is often not connected to this growth in size is the increasing level of estradiol in many men. Also, men begin to gain some weight, fat to be more specific, around the waist at this same time. This may well be associated with low levels of progesterone, sometimes thought of as a female hormone…but it is not. In men as in women, one function performed by progesterone is to balance insulin. When this balance is upset by declining levels of progesterone, the human body is more likely to store excess blood sugar in fat cells.

These fat cells contain a substance known as aromatase, which can convert testosterone into estradiol. Estradiol, in turn, is known to cause cancer in the women's tissues that have the same fetal origins as the male prostate. This means that cancer of the prostate may not be a simple lowering of testosterone levels or the rise of estradiol levels. It also probably includes the decreasing progesterone level as an element of the process.

There is a commonly held misconception that testosterone is the cause of prostate cancer. (If this were actually true, we would expect to see many more cases of prostate cancer among young men. But this is not so!) Since low testosterone is associated with an increased risk of prostate cancer, the above discussion would lead one to believe that the process that results in some or many such prostate cancers is much more complex.

In summary, decreasing progesterone leads to increased insulin levels. This then encourages an increase in abdominal fat cells that, utilizing aromatase, converts at least some testosterone to estradiol, thereby increasing estradiol levels and further lowering testosterone available to the body. This increase in estradiol then may be the ultimate bad actor.

> Estradiol, not testosterone, may be the ultimate cause of prostate cancer.

If this problem is a complex reaction to hormones increasing and decreasing, where would a solution start? An obvious first step would be to treat the lack of progesterone with a physiologic dose to bring that back into a healthy level. This should assist in lowering available body fat and reduce the conversion of testosterone to estradiol.

Adding chrysin to a testosterone transdermal cream may be part of the answer as well. Chrysin, an aromatase inhibitor, may help reduce the conversion of testosterone to estradiol by interrupting that aspect of the problem. Zinc, an important supplement in maintaining prostate health, also can act as an aromatase inhibitor.

If these measures still do not reduce estradiol to an appropriate level, the use of a drug such as anastrozole might be helpful. It should also be noted that the body can make testosterone from progesterone. It might be possible in some cases to not only lower fat cell actions but raise available testosterone with progesterone treatment alone. As we note throughout this book, however, never forget that you are an experiment of one when it comes to assessing the impact of hormones on your health. What works for someone else, may not work for you.

The above discussion includes a complex process that may lead to prostate cancer. Any procedures put in place to maintain a healthy prostate or to assist in treating cancer should be carefully monitored by a trained physician. Since the use of bio-identical hormones to address men's health is a relatively new field of specialization, it is recommended that you find a physician specifically trained to use these products and related drugs and supplements.

The PSA (prostate specific antigen) test is commonly used to assess the risk of prostate cancer in a patient. It may be of value in some instances but is all-too-often associated with false positives. Also, one study found that relatively low PSA values in combination with low testosterone was not predictive of good prostate health; of those with PSA values less than 4, 15-30% of patients had biopsy-proven prostate cancer.

It should be noted that active sexual behavior within 48-72 hours of a PSA test may result in a false positive. So those anticipating a PSA test within that time frame should keep their bodies and minds free of sexual actions of any kind. There are also some physicians who worry that biopsies of the prostate may in fact spread cancer cells if they are present. This argues for a second PSA test to verify initial results before moving forward with more invasive treatment.

So, what is one to do? The best action, hopefully taken early, is to maintain good prostate health by keeping related hormone levels at appropriate, healthy levels to prevent problems from beginning. Getting rid of that abdominal fat would also be a good start; proper supplements as indicated by testing, diet and exercise should work together with those healthy hormones.

12

Exercise and Diet

We all know that exercise and diet are key factors in maintaining a healthy body that is capable of addressing the challenges of today. Both help the body to adapt to a stressful environment that starts almost with awakening. What we eat, how much of it we eat, and how we use the potential energy provided by food will determine much of our health. This becomes more and more evident with age as the youthful hormones slowly decline.

There seem to be almost as many diets as there are people on the planet. How does one pick a diet that is appropriate to oneself? The answer would have to be "carefully" and with full knowledge of the needs of the particular body in question. We are all—with the possible exception of identical siblings—genetically unique. Our bodies (and our minds) will respond to our environments in a unique manner. These unique responses will demand specific things from our diet to support appropriate reactions.

As an example, the body responds to a stressful event with the "fight or flight" response. In this moment of perceived crisis the body makes almost instantaneous changes, driven in large part by our hormones, to respond to a challenging situation. When the event concludes, we readapt to a less stressful situation. Certain foods can be helpful if we are constantly exposed to this type of change.

A diet designed for today is probably similar to that on which early humans depended, one long on fruit and vegetables and supplemented with animal protein. We will leave the debate about organic foods for another time, but the fresher the food we eat, the better it tends to be for us. Keep thinking what those early humans ate, and you will probably remain close to on target.

Beware that low-fat diets may not be that good for your hormone health. Without enough fat, your body probably will not be able to make enough testosterone, DHEA and cortisol—all important to good health in the proper quantities.

And water! Plain water is great for us and an average of two quarts a day should keep everything properly moist. If you exercise heavily, you may need to increase this level to ensure that you do not become dehydrated. It would be a good idea to avoid many of the exercise drinks as they often contain unneeded salts and caffeine. The latter can be particularly dangerous in large doses even though it may give one a sense of energy for the moment.

The things to avoid in your diet would be those, again, not common to early humans. Grains, as an example, were not added to the human diet until civilizations began to form around farmers' fields. They don't need to be totally ignored, but minimal amounts are probably enough. Many humans are not adapted to digest dairy products, legumes and nuts...even though they can be valuable sources of nutrients. Yeast, as commonly present in breads and related products, may lead to fungal infections in our digestive tracts, which, in turn, may lead to fluctuating hormone levels as well as some allergies, bloated feelings and gas.

Coffee, tea and other caffeine drinks are diuretic. In large quantities they can cause dehydration. A large amount of coffee to start your day may also initiate the "fight or flight" response noted earlier. Keep your consumption to two cups or less and you will be fine in that regard. If you have a choice of decaffeinated varieties, take them instead. Herbal teas may not be diuretic and might also be an alternative.

Alcohol would require at least a chapter to properly discuss, but moderation here is always recommended. There are benefits to moderate consumption, but there are always the dangers of overconsumption and the yeast-friendly nature of fermented products.

Chasing every passing great diet, no matter who has endorsed it and had wonderful results, is not healthy. If you change your eating pattern, be careful to assure that you have not chosen something that your body cannot tolerate. Remember that we are all an experiment of one. (It wouldn't be bad to have a physician's guidance here if this is critical to making you return to a healthy lifestyle.)

And then there is exercise. We all seem to recognize that we need more of it and benefit from a regular dose. With the advent of modern work-saving devices we now get significantly less exercise than our ancestors. Instead of walking two miles to school in the snow (uphill both ways), we ride in a car, often for only a few blocks. We work long distances from home and spend a lot of time riding in both directions. We sit behind a desk for the better part of a day or drive from work site to work site.

Few would argue against a regular exercise program, but many would admit that they do not follow a regular routine that builds muscle and endurance. If you are one of the many, you should not immediately leap into a program designed for twenty-year-olds and expect dynamic results. What you want, instead, is a moderate program that avoids injuries while slowly building a healthy, strong body.

And if you were a world-class athlete twenty years ago, don't feel you can jump back into that routine without taking the time to start over. Get the guidance of a trainer who works regularly with normal people, those with moderate goals and a need to proceed slowly. Rapid progress followed by injury after injury will get you nowhere.

The author would recommend a combination of aerobic and non-aerobic exercise, the former to build a strong cardiovascular system and the latter to build strong muscles (and bones). If you haven't exercised recently, start your program with a physical to ensure that your body can support the training you desire. If you need hormone treatments, ensure that the hormones are achieving their proper levels before you get too strenuous with the exercise. Start moderately, perhaps walking or exercising in a swimming pool. Three great exercise areas are running, swimming and bicycle riding; they all provide great benefits for your cardiovascular system. However, they all require proper preparation.

Runners should start slow and taper off. Running short intervals and then walking the rest of the way or walking distances over time is a great way to start. Swimmers must be satisfied with gradual gains until they build the right sets of muscles. Bikers need all the proper safety equipment and training as well as a safe place to ride. It does no good to be in great shape and encounter a large moving vehicle.

Before starting to exercise, it is recommended that you stretch the muscles that will be used. The same is true after a good exercise period. Slow stretches are best as you can injure yourself overdoing a stretch just as you can injure yourself exercising. Self-massage of sore areas can be helpful as can observing the RICE methodology for dealing with muscular injuries: rest, ice, compression and elevation.

Start exercise programs slowly after you are assured by a physician that you are in appropriate good health.

Beware of medical help that suggests pain medication; ask how to cure the underlying problem. As an example, tendonitis is often the reflection of a muscle injury on the opposite side of the joint where the tendon inflammation occurs. Look for a sore area and use massage to work on that spot. Allowing the muscle to move freely may often eliminate the pain and prevent a more serious injury later. A trained massage specialist can be very helpful here.

You now have balanced your hormones, eaten properly and exercised your body. What else could there possibly be?

13

Nutritional Supplements

Some people may not need them. Some people may need quite a few. What is recommend is to select only those you need and to take them according to the recommendations of a medical professional. Simply stuffing yourself with every supplement that knocks on your door is not going to ensure good health. In fact, overdosing can present its own problems.

Discussed here are a few key supplements that should be considered. It is not a complete list, and it is not designed for everyone. Remember that you are an experiment of one and you should know that what you are putting into your body is needed by your body. Let's touch on a few key items.

First, let's talk about vitamins. Is a multiple vitamin tablet taken as described by the manufacturer good for your health? Possibly! What you should know is that it will not usually hurt you unless you are taking other vitamins separately and they contribute to an overdose. What no one can say without testing and consulting with a patient is exactly which vitamins might be of greatest value. If eating habits are erratic or the intake of fresh fruit and vegetables is limited, a multiple vitamin might avoid a deficiency problem.

For the rest of us, we might want to target areas where supplements are known to have a specific and positive impact. As an example, Vitamin B_{12}, magnesium and Coenzyme Q10 (CoQ10) are known to be particularly valuable in addressing fatigue. The latter is especially valuable to muscle health and may be, thus, of great value to your heart. With a healthier heart, you can expect greater blood flow with the same amount of effort. This allows the blood to distribute other nutrients throughout the body more efficiently.

Are you under constant stress? Vitamin B_6, calcium and magnesium may be valuable. There are a number of nutrients that may assist in combating depression, and these include thiamin, folic acid, Vitamin C, calcium, zinc and potassium. If these or other symptoms are present, you should do some simple research to identify all that may be appropriate. It is recommended that you consult with a knowledgeable healthcare provider for additional and specific advice. It also would be a good idea to shy away from commercial information sources intent on selling products as a first intention rather than providing unbiased guidance.

One of the great undiscovered secrets may be Vitamin D3, regarded by some as a hormone or pre-hormone. This is available without prescription and may have a benefit of helping the human immune system to resist certain viruses. The recommended daily allowance (RDA) is a relatively low 600 international units (ius) per day. One study found the vitamin to be safe to levels as high as 100,000 ius per day; that same article recommended that takers use 15,000 ius per day as a dosage. At this level many of those vulnerable to colds, sore throats and possibly pneumonia may develop strong resistance. Upon encountering the beginning symptoms, increasing the dosage significantly for several days may kill the attacking virus. Research here is incomplete but compelling.

This chapter is not designed to provide comprehensive information regarding nutritional elements, only to point out that the human body sometimes needs more than our diets can provide. Given the few examples provided, we would expect the reader to do some additional research. Several of the books at the end of the last chapter may prove helpful, but, as always, professional assistance is recommended when available so as to supplement individual research.

Remember that you are a unique human being and should spend some time researching what your body needs rather than taking supplements just because they might provide some benefit.

One last note! If you have decided to take a statin drug to lower cholesterol, you should always take CoQ10 as a supplement as those drugs deplete the body of naturally acquired supplies. If you take a bisphosphonate drug (Boniva, Fosamax, etc.) to address bone density, you should take additional calcium. This calcium is not for building healthy bones but is for other uses in the body; this class of drugs stops the normal removal of old bone (calcium) for use in maintaining other healthy organs. Since the normal bone healing and building process is artificially interrupted, calcium will not be properly absorbed by the bones. This is discussed further in Chapter 6.

14

Finding Medical Help

If you have a family physician who knows the value of hormone treatments, you are among the lucky few. Most doctors working within the large healthcare organizations are either not knowledgeable or do not have access to the bio-identical hormones that are so important to many of the concepts voiced in this book. You should not accept synthetic products that are not bio-identical where the latter are available if the ideas in this book have gotten your interest.

The best source of information would be friends who have already discovered the value of hormone balancing as combined with proper nutrition and exercise. Although hormone issues can arise at any age, friends who have passed 40 years of age would be those of most value to many of us in evaluating options.

Without friends to guide us, contacting a compounding pharmacy may provide some recommendations as to doctors with whom they work. Since compounding pharmacies are the source of many of the bio-identical products that support this natural approach to health, they regularly work with doctors who prescribe treatments designed for specific individuals by their doctors.

> Compounding pharmacies may be able to provide the names of local doctors with whom they work to supply bio-identical products.

Of course there is always the internet. You must be careful to evaluate medical recommendations obtained there carefully as this is an emerging specialty, one of "anti-aging medicine." There are always a few opportunists who prey on those who have difficulty recognizing high quality professional services from clever marketing.

In the back of Susanne Somers' book *Breakthrough: Eight Steps to Wellness* is an excellent list of resources. Although the author does not agree with all the advice she provides in her books, she is definitely on the right track.

15

Last Comments

From the beginning of this book it has been noted that your health is an experiment of one. Each person is unique and requires appropriate, individual attention. You need to be in charge of each step as you do your best to maintain good health while you age. This book advocates the achievement of hormone levels that are healthy, not just normal for your age. And these levels must be determined under the guidance of trained healthcare professionals.

It is strongly recommended that everyone have a baseline of healthy hormones established and then monitor levels into the future as "things change." You may be under more or less stress, begin or end an exercise routine, change your diet or move to a new external environment. All these can influence your hormone levels.

And when should these healthy hormone levels be established? Ideally, we would all have a complete panel of tests when we are at our healthiest. This often means in our early to mid-thirties. This age for testing will often not be possible as treatment may well begin long after that age. Instead, once you have established levels that provide the best health for you, take note of those values. This may be a reasonable alternative and provide an excellent starting point for long-term treatment.

If we live long enough, many of us will encounter post-traumatic stress disorder (PTSD). Often associated with military personnel who encounter terrible events in a wartime environment, such common events as a freeway accident or the sudden death of a close friend or life partner may bring on the symptoms of PTSD.

These symptoms, which include persistently re-experiencing the event, increased arousal or avoidance of things associated with the causal event, are often treated by psychiatric professionals. Since these types of stressful events are known to cause hormonal responses, we would recommend that treatment begin with the development of a hormone test panel to see where hormones may require supplementation. Once the physical aspects of body chemistry have been remedied, psychiatric or psychological techniques should be much more effective.

Now that your hormones have been balanced to healthy levels, and you are supplemented, exercised and eaten the best you can:

Gentlemen: Start your engines!

And

ROAR LIKE A LION!

Acknowledgement

The author acknowledges the emerging field of anti-aging medicine and the innovative and pioneering doctors and researchers dedicated to the development of this specialized field. Moving the healthcare system focused on the management of diseases to one pointed toward maintaining good health will be a slow and painful transition. In this new paradigm, patients will need to be more actively engaged and knowledgeable so as to ask for the best options available and provide the most accurate histories to their healthcare providers. The author hopes that this book will provide a small push in this new direction.

References (Some Books Worth Reading)

1. Thierry Hertogue (2002). *The Hormone Solution: Stay Younger Longer*.

2. John R. Lee & Virginia Hopkins (2006). *Dr. John Lee's Hormone Balance Made Simple*.

3. Edward Lichten (2007). *Textbook of Bio-Identical Hormones*.

4. Chris D. Meletis & Sara G. Wood (2009). *His Change of Life*.

5. Michael Platt (2007). *The Miracle of Bio-Identical Hormones*.

6. Jonathan Wright & Lane Lenard (2010). *Stay Young & Sexy with Bio-Identical Hormone Replacement: The Science Explained*.

7. Jonathan Wright & Lane Lenard (2006). *Maximize Your Vitality & Potency For Men Over 40.*

More References (Some Technical Ones)

1. Bain, J. (2001). Andropause: Testosterone replacement therapy for aging men. *Canadian Family Physician 47*: 91-97.

2. Bassil, N., Alkaade, S. & Morley, J.E. (2009). The benefits and risks of testosterone replacement therapy: A review. *Therapeutics and Clinical Risk Management*; *9*: 427-448.

3. Carruthers, M. (2007, March). Time for international action on treating testosterone deficiency syndrome. *The Aging Male*; *12(1):* 21-28.

4. Feldman, HA, Longcope, C. & Derby, C.A. (2002). "Age trends in the level of serum testosterone and other hormones in middle-aged men: Longitudinal results from the Massachusetts male aging study." *Journal of Clinical Endocrinological Metabolism*: *87, pp.* 589-598.

5. Geddes, L. (2008). One in five men get the 'andropause': Could hormone replacement therapy become commonplace in older men? *New Scientist, 200* (8).

6. Laughlin, G.A., Barrett-Connor, E. & Bergstrom, J. (2008). Low serum testosterone and mortality in older men. *Journal of Clinical Endocrinology & Metabolism*; *93*: 68-75.

7. Morales, A. (2008). The use of hormonal therapy in "andropause": The pro side. *Journal of the Canadian Urological Association*; *2(1):* 43-45.

8. Rajfer, J. (2003). Decreased testosterone in the aging male: summary and conclusions. *Reviews in Urology*; *5(suppl 1):* S49-S50.

9. Shores, M.M., Matsumoto, A.M. Sloan, K. & Kivlahan, D. (2006). Low serum testosterone and mortality in male veterans. *Archives of Internal Medicine*; *166*: 1660-1665.

About the Author

Port R. (Bob) Martin, EdD, has had a long interest in medical subjects and physical fitness, starting when he began reading medically related books at age 10. After a number of careers in government and private sector organizations, he began researching bio-identical hormones in 2009 as a possible solution to his growing fatigue and recurring encounters with cold viruses and pneumonia. He has personally tested most of the recommendations included in this book as well as discussing them with a number of medical experts. He lives and works in San Diego, CA, where he moved after growing up in Walla Walla, WA.